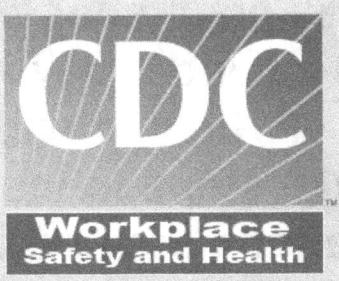

I0415782

Evaluation of Heat and Carbon Monoxide Exposures to Border Protection Officers at Ports of Entry

Chad Dowell, MS, CIH

Judith Eisenberg, MD, MS

Health Hazard Evaluation Report
HETA 2005-0215-3099
Department of Homeland Security
U.S. Customs and Border Protection
El Paso, Texas
December 2009

Department of Health and Human Services
Centers for Disease Control and Prevention

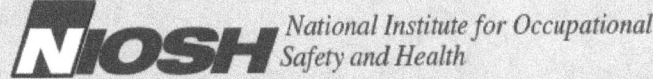

National Institute for Occupational Safety and Health

CONTENTS

ABBREVIATIONS

ACGIH®	American Conference of Governmental Industrial Hygienists
BEI®	Biological exposure limit
bpm	Beats per minute
BUN	Blood urea nitrogen
CBP	Customs and Border Protection
CBT	Core body temperature
CFR	Code of Federal Regulations
CO	Carbon monoxide
COHb	Carboxyhemoglobin
HHE	Health hazard evaluation
IDLH	Immediately dangerous to life and health
kcal/hour	Kilocalories per hour
mEq/L	Milliequivalents per liter
mg/dL	Milligrams per deciliter
mosm/L	Millimoles per liter
NIOSH	National Institute for Occupational Safety and Health
OEL	Occupational exposure limit
OSHA	Occupational Safety and Health Administration
PBZ	Personal breathing zone
PEL	Permissible exposure limit
ppm	Parts per million
RAL	Recommended action limit
REL	Recommended exposure limit
STEL	Short term exposure limit
TLV®	Threshold limit value
TWA	Time-weighted average
WBGT	Wet bulb globe temperature
WEEL	Workplace environmental exposure level

Highlights of the NIOSH Health Hazard Evaluation

The National Institute for Occupational Safety and Health (NIOSH) received a union request for a health hazard evaluation at the Customs and Border Protection (CBP) ports of entry in El Paso, Texas. The request concerned CBP officers' work in hot environments and potential exposure to carbon monoxide from vehicle exhaust.

What NIOSH Did

- We made a site visit in August and September 2005.
- We talked with management and union officials about the working conditions in outdoor vehicle inspection areas.
- We measured officers' exposure to heat and humidity in outdoor vehicle inspection areas.
- We measured officers' exposure to carbon monoxide in outdoor vehicle inspection areas.
- We talked to officers about their work environment, work practices, and work-related concerns.

What NIOSH Found

- Officers were not exposed to excessive heat at the time of this evaluation; however, heat exposure can be greater during the summer.
- No formal heat stress management program was in place.
- Officers did not report symptoms related to heat exposure.
- Officers' carbon monoxide exposures were over the peak limit but not the full-shift exposure limit.
- None of the officers exceeded the recommended limit for carboxyhemoglobin, an indicator of carbon monoxide exposure.

What Managers Can Do

- Start a formal heat stress management program.
- Allow officers to take unscheduled breaks away from the hot environment if needed. Signs of excess heat exposure include weakness, nausea, confusion, excessive tiredness, or irritability.
- Develop a hazard communication program. The program should address working in hot environments and working around vehicle exhaust.
- Continue to rotate officers between primary and secondary vehicle inspection areas.
- Monitor officers' exposure to carbon monoxide.
- Require that vehicles be turned off during inspection of the undercarriage.

HIGHLIGHTS OF THE NIOSH HEALTH HAZARD EVALUATION (CONTINUED)

What Employees Can Do

- Tell your supervisor if you feel weak, nauseated, excessively fatigued, confused, and/or irritable due to the heat.

- Drink plenty of fluids.

- Require drivers to turn off their vehicle when inspecting the undercarriage.

- Do not place your head near the vehicle's exhaust while the vehicle is running.

SUMMARY

On April 22, 2005, NIOSH received a union request asking NIOSH to evaluate heat stress and CO exposures for CBP officers working in the outdoor vehicle inspection areas at the CBP ports of entry in El Paso, Texas. The request indicated that some officers had experienced heat cramps and heat exhaustion. In response, NIOSH investigators monitored heat stress, heat strain, and CO in air and exhaled breath on August 29–September 2, 2005, at the Bridge of the Americas and Paso del Norte ports of entry in El Paso, Texas.

Heat stress and strain measurements collected during this evaluation showed that CBP officers in the outdoor vehicle inspection areas were not exposed to heat stress over the occupational recommendations. Officers have the potential for high peak CO exposures. Full shift CO exposures and %COHb were below occupational exposure limits. We recommend that CBP implement administrative controls to minimize the potential for heat strain and reduce CO exposures.

At the time of our evaluation we found that officers working in the outdoor vehicle inspection areas were not exposed to heat stress that exceeded NIOSH and ACGIH recommendations. None of the officers monitored for heat strain showed signs of excessive heat stress exposure. However, environmental temperatures are often warmer in El Paso than they were on the days of our evaluations. Higher temperatures would increase the likelihood that occupational heat stress recommendations could be exceeded and that employees could be at increased risk of heat strain.

The NIOSH recommended exposure limit ceiling for CO was exceeded for some of the officers working in the outdoor vehicle inspection areas. This REL was exceeded when the officers inspected the vehicle's undercarriage near the exhaust pipe. None of the officers monitored exceeded the full shift TWA occupational exposure limits for CO or the limits for COHb.

Investigators recommended creating a formal heat stress management program that includes information on heat acclimatization and heat stress prevention. Management should monitor environmental heat exposure and develop criteria for heat alerts. Investigators also recommended turning off vehicles in primary inspection lanes, creating a hazard communication program for working around vehicle exhaust, continuing to use officer rotation schedules, and periodically monitoring officers' CO exposures.

Keywords: NAICS 928110 (National Security), heat stress, heat strain, carbon monoxide, vehicle exhaust, vehicle inspection, immigration, customs and border protection

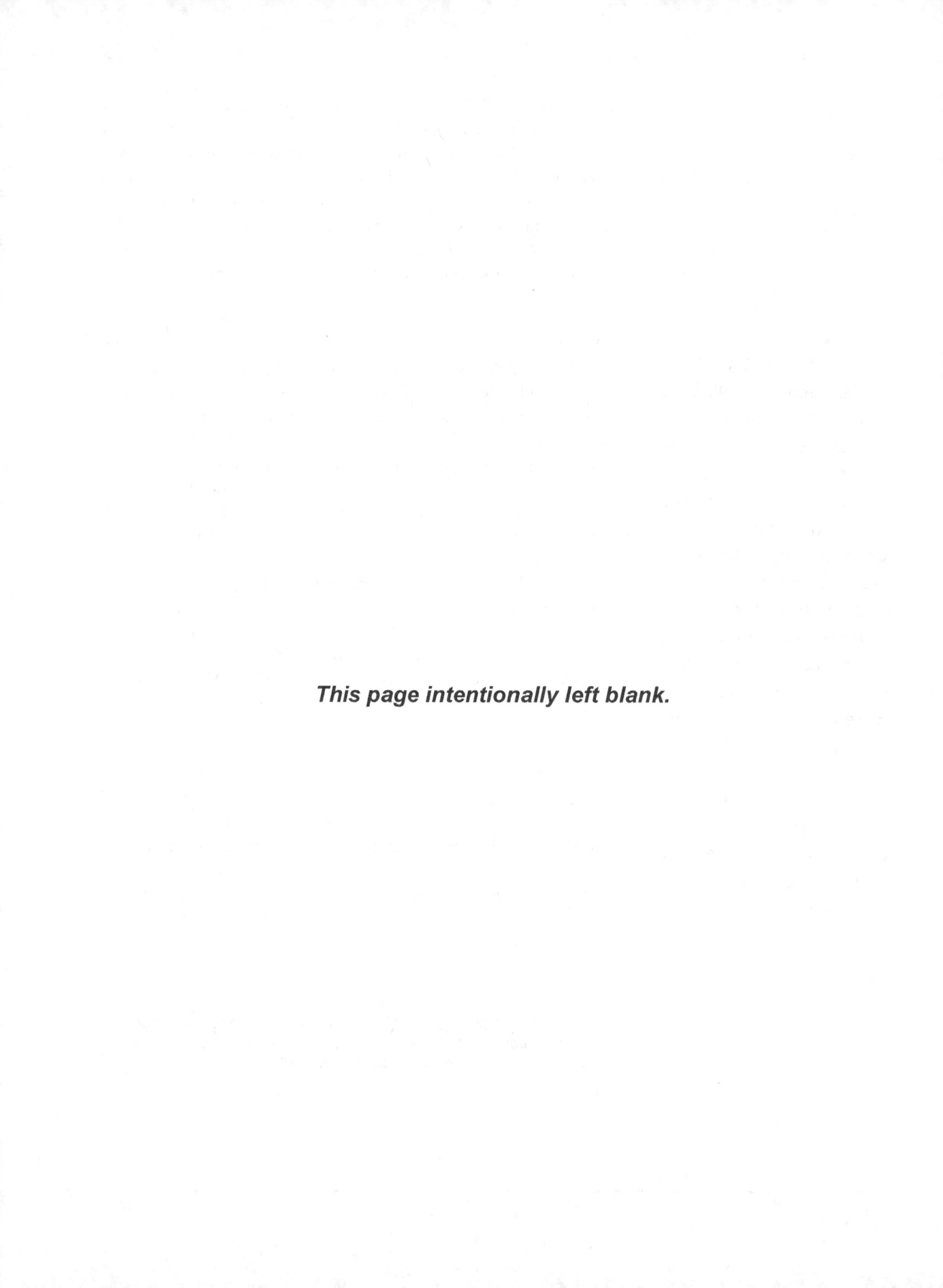

This page intentionally left blank.

INTRODUCTION

On April 22, 2005, NIOSH received a request from the American Federation of Government Employees for an HHE at the CBP ports of entry in El Paso, Texas. The HHE request asked NIOSH to evaluate heat stress and CO exposures for CBP officers working in the outdoor vehicle inspection areas. The request indicated that some CBP officers had experienced heat cramps and heat exhaustion. In response, NIOSH investigators monitored heat strain, heat stress, CO in air, and COHb on August 29–September 2, 2005, at the Bridge of the Americas and Paso del Norte ports of entry.

El Paso has three ports of entry from Mexico: Bridge of the Americas, Paso del Norte, and Ysleta. All three ports of entry operate 24 hours a day with CBP officers inspecting incoming vehicles and pedestrian traffic. Bridge of the Americas is the largest of the three ports of entry with 14 primary vehicle inspection lanes staffed by approximately 28 CBP officers per 8-hour shift. The Paso del Norte port of entry has 9 primary vehicle inspection lanes, and Ysleta has 12 lanes, although typically only 6 of the 12 lanes are open for vehicular inspection due to limited demand. Each port of entry has a secondary vehicle inspection area. Both the primary and secondary vehicle inspection areas at all three ports of entry are covered with a canopy roof.

All vehicular traffic enters the ports of entry through one of the primary inspection lanes. During the primary inspection, the driver's credentials are checked, and the vehicle is inspected. CBP officers often use a hand-held mirror and mallet to check the undercarriage of the vehicle, a practice requiring them to bend down near the exhaust pipe. Although the CBP officer can require the driver to turn off the vehicle during the inspection, many CBP officers do not require this because the driver may be unable to restart the vehicle, thus blocking the lane. If a more thorough inspection is necessary, cars are directed to the secondary inspection area and turned off.

The inspection booths at the three ports of entry are similar in size and configuration and are provided outdoor air from overhead ducts. This air can be heated but not cooled. Directly outside the inspection booth, overhead air showers blow outdoor air downward in the area where CBP officers perform most of their duties. Each primary inspection lane has one CBP officer, while the secondary inspection area has multiple CBP officers. The CBP officers' job responsibilities require them to work mostly outside the inspection booths except when they are recording and entering

INTRODUCTION
(CONTINUED)

information into a computer. The inspection booths have sliding glass doors that face the inspection lane, but these are frequently left open to facilitate access between the inside of the inspection booth and the vehicles. The secondary inspection area is covered by a canopy. CBP officers rotate between the primary inspection lanes and the secondary inspection area throughout their work shift with a 30-minute lunch break. All shifts are 8 hours long, but employees have options for voluntary overtime.

Beneath the secondary inspection canopy area, fans mounted on the canopy roof provide dilution ventilation. The CBP officers control these fans. None of the ports of entry is equipped with local exhaust ventilation systems for controlling automobile exhaust in the primary or secondary inspection areas.

ASSESSMENT

Heat stress, heat strain, and CO exposures were assessed at the Bridge of the Americas and Paso del Norte, the two busiest El Paso ports of entry. These two ports of entry perform similar vehicular inspection operations with only minor differences in the neighboring buildings and the number of inspection lanes. The Ysleta port of entry was not evaluated because of the limited number of cars passing through. This decision was made in consultation with the union and CBP management.

To evaluate heat stress conditions, eight WBGT measurements were collected in the primary and secondary inspection lanes and inside the primary inspection booths and head house. For the heat strain evaluation, 24 participants volunteered to be monitored for physiological responses to the conditions of the work environment. Twenty-three CBP officers were monitored over one shift and one CBP officer over two shifts, for a total of 25 individual measurements. CBT, heart rate, preshift and postshift weight, and blood chemistries were measured for each participant. Blood chemistries monitored included serum sodium, potassium, chloride, BUN, and glucose. Hemoglobin and hematocrit were also measured. Thirty-three participants, including 24 CBP officers involved in the heat strain monitoring and 9 additional CBP officers, volunteered to be monitored for CO exposure. All 33 participants wore PBZ CO monitors, and 28 had their preshift and postshift COHb levels evaluated by exhaled breath measurements. A detailed discussion of the methods used for this evaluation is available in Appendix A, and a detailed discussion of the applicable occupational exposure limits is available in Appendix B.

Heat Stress

Individual WBGT measurements are reported in Tables 1 and 2. The highest WBGT reading between Bridge of the Americas and Paso del Norte was 82.9°F, with dry bulb temperatures averaging between 82.5°F and 85.1°F. In the head house (the CBP officers' break room) the highest WBGT reading was 71.4°F, with a dry bulb temperature of 78.1°F. At the time of this evaluation the dry bulb (ambient) temperatures were cooler than usual for that time of year [NOAA 2000]. These cooler ambient temperatures likely lessened the heat stress hazard in the inspection areas during the week of our evaluation.

Table 1. Heat stress measurements, Bridge of the Americas, August 30–31, 2005

Monitoring Location	Sample Time	Temperature (°F)	
		WBGT (range)	Dry Bulb (range)
Inside inspection booth of lane 5	0903–1600	72.4°F (66.4°F–77.8°F)	83.6°F (74.7°F–93.1°F)
Secondary inspection area*	0900–1601	71.2°F (65.1°F–81.8°F)	85.1°F (73.7°F–96.5°F)
Head house†	0914–1208‡	59.5°F (53.9°F–71.4°F)	64.5°F (58.1°F–78.1°F)
Outside booth of lane 5*	0902–1600	71.8°F (65.7°F–77.6°F)	84.9°F (74.8°F–96.4°F)

* Outdoor measurement
† Indoor WBGT value, representative of where some CBP officers take their breaks.
‡ Monitor turned off by a CBP officer overnight.

Table 2. Heat stress measurements, Paso del Norte, September 1–2, 2005

Monitoring Location	Sample Time	Temperature (°F)	
		WBGT (range)	Dry Bulb (range)
Inside inspection booth of lane 5	0854–1555	70.1°F (65.1°F–78.2°F)	77.0°F (71.6°F–89.5°F)
Secondary inspection area*	0841–1559	70.9°F (64.2°F–82.9°F)	82.5 °F (69.6°F–98.2°F)
Head house†	0851–1601	68.2°F (66.0°F–70.9°F)	76.7°F (74.0°F–81.4°F)
Outside booth of lane 5*	0846–0402	71.2°F (64.1°F–77.6°F)	82.7°F (69.4°F–95.4°F)

* Outdoor measurement
† Indoor WBGT value, representative of where some CBP officers take their breaks

The metabolic rates for the CBP officers working in the primary and secondary inspection areas were estimated between 120 and 156 kcal/hour. Because the CBP officers wore a uniform (long sleeve shirt and pants), no clothing-adjustment factors were added to the WBGT measurements. The metabolic rates and the WBGT data listed in Table 1 and 2 were compared to the NIOSH and ACGIH heat stress recommendations. Neither the NIOSH nor the ACGIH heat stress recommendations were exceeded for any of the CBP officers.

Heat Strain

A total of 24 participants completed a short heat stress questionnaire. The median age of the participating CBP officers was 37 years. The median duration of employment at the two El Paso ports of entry was 3 years, with range of 3 months to 15 years. None of the officers gave positive responses for the question regarding "any problems with heat exposure in the past year."

Individual heat strain measurements are reported in Table 3. All except two CBP officers were considered acclimatized to their work environment; two CBP officers reported they had just returned from a 4-day absence. The average CBT ranged from 98.71°F to 100.2°F, below the 101.3°F for medically fit, heat-acclimatized employees. The ACGIH recommendation for unacclimatized employees of 100.4°F was not exceeded for either of the two unacclimatized CBP officers. None of the CBP officers developed signs of heat strain when compared to the ACGIH recommendation for acclimatized employees.

Participants' heart rates did not exceed the ACGIH recommendation of 180 bpm minus the employee's age. Due to instrument error, no heart rate measurements were collected on September 2, 2005.

Body weight changes over the participants' shift ranged from a 1% loss to a 2% gain, with an average of a 0.2% gain. None of the CBP officers tested had a body weight change of more than the ACGIH recommendation of a 1.5% loss.

Table 3. Individual physiological measurements

Date	Sampling Period	Average CBT (°F)	Average Heart Rate (bpm)	Body Weight Change (%)
Bridge of the Americas				
August 30, 2005	0823–1333*	98.71	74	0.0
	0833–1351*	99.29	50	−0.2
	0836–1339	†	77	−0.3
	0850–1403	99.03	96	−1
	0841–1535	99.41	88	0.8
August 31, 2005	0722–1505	99.21	‡	2
	0757–1547	99.00	84	1
	0803–1544	99.44	73	0.0
	0720–1333	100.2	70	2
	0852–1516	99.54	96	0.0
	0816–1340	99.91	83	0.5
	0929–1519	99.72	91	0.0
Paso del Norte				
September 1, 2005	0729–1333	99.94	99	0.9
	0813–1328	99.72	97	0.2
	0817–1607	99.68	60	−0.9
	0719–1446	99.36	†	−0.8
	0829–1539	99.72	84	1
	0719–1446	99.36	74	−0.4
	0854–1547	†	84	0.6
	0918–1349	98.75	†	0.9
September 2, 2005	0715–1534	99.50	†	−0.3
	0736–1332	99.28	†	0.0
	0840–1526	99.25	†	−0.7
	0900–1328	99.63	†	−0.3
	0908–1528	99.51	†	−0.7

* Unacclimatized CBP officer
† No data collected
‡ No data reported due to instrument error

Most serum electrolytes, including serum sodium, potassium, chloride, BUN, and glucose, were within normal limits for both preshift and postshift testing. The reference range for serum sodium is 135–145 mEq/L. A corrected serum sodium was calculated for those participants with elevated serum glucose levels because high serum glucose (> 100 mg/dL) can cause falsely low measurements of serum sodium. Once the corrected sodium was calculated for those participants, all participants had preshift and postshift serum sodium levels within the reference range. The serum osmolality reference range is 275–290 mosm/L; the formula used for its calculation incorporates the values of serum sodium, BUN, and glucose. Aside from those participants who had elevated serum glucose levels, all other preshift and postshift serum osmolalities fell within the reference range.

No participants had a past medical history of diabetes, nor did any of the participants with elevated glucose readings report symptoms consistent with hyperglycemia such as polyuria (frequent urination), polydipsia (excessive thirst), headache, abdominal pain or blurred vision.

Carbon Monoxide

Full shift CO exposures ranged up to 22 ppm, with an average concentration of 8 ppm; none exceeded the OSHA PEL of 50 ppm, the NIOSH REL of 35 ppm, or the ACGIH TLV of 25 ppm. Peak CO exposures greater than 999 ppm (the maximum limit of the CO monitor) were measured on 14 participants; these concentrations exceeded the NIOSH recommended ceiling limit of 200 ppm. CBP officers reported noticing their monitors responding to these peak CO concentrations when they were inspecting near a vehicle's exhaust pipe.

When analyzing results for COHb, different reference ranges are used for nonsmokers and smokers because smokers generally have higher baseline COHb levels. For all the nonsmoker employees we measured in this evaluation, the average preshift COHb level was 0.86%, and the average postshift level was 0.88%, an increase of 2.3%. For all smokers, the average preshift COHb level was 3.0%, and the average postshift level was 2.7%, representing a decrease of 8.8%. None of the nonsmoking participants exceeded the ACGIH BEI for CO of 3.5% COHb at the end of shift. All of the participants were within or below the World Health Organization's reference ranges for COHb of 1%–2% for nonsmokers and 3%–8% for smokers.

DISCUSSION

At the time of our evaluation, CBP had no formal program in place for ensuring that the CBP officers were protected from heat stress and CO exposure. A few administrative controls were in place, though not intended for health reasons. For example, a work schedule required the CBP officers to rotate from the primary inspection lanes to the secondary inspection areas every 30 minutes. This rotation policy, however, was implemented for security reasons to prevent any CBP officer from being able to tell anyone where they would be working at any specific time. CBP officers in the primary inspection lanes were also given the option of requiring specific drivers to turn off the vehicle during the inspection if it was in a state of poor repair or using a poor quality fuel. However, many of the CBP officers reported that they did not ask drivers to turn off their vehicles because the drivers may not have been able to restart them.

One medication taken by some participants that could potentially affect heat stress responses was Toprol XL, an extended release form of a beta blocker. One participant reported being treated for hypertension but could not recall the type of medication. Beta blockers are medications that directly depress heart rate and are commonly used in patients with cardiovascular atherosclerotic disease and hypertension.

Those individuals with mild elevations of serum glucose (between 100-200 mg/dL) were advised to follow up with their personal physicians within a week to have their blood sugar retested. Two participants with serum glucose levels over 200 mg/dL were given copies of their results and encouraged to make an appointment with their personal physicians.

CONCLUSIONS

CBP officers working in the primary and secondary vehicle inspection areas were not exposed to heat stress and strain that exceeded the occupational recommendations during the NIOSH evaluation. However, ambient temperatures may be warmer at other times during the summer, raising the potential for heat stress and strain [NOAA 2000].

The NIOSH recommended ceiling limit for CO was exceeded for some of the CBP officers. These CBP officers' peak CO exposures lasted less than a minute and were associated with inspection

CONCLUSIONS

activities near a vehicle exhaust pipe. However, no CBP officer monitored for CO exceeded a full shift OEL, and none of the participants exceeded the ACGIH BEI for %COHb.

RECOMMENDATIONS

The following recommendations help identify potential heat stress and strain risks and help limit heat-related illnesses in CBP officers.

1. Develop a heat-acclimatization program to decrease the risk of heat-related disorders. Such a program involves exposing CBP officers to hot work environments for progressively longer periods. NIOSH recommends that CBP officers who have had previous experience in jobs where heat levels are high enough to produce heat stress (CBT and heart rate increase, but do not exceed recommended levels) should work in the environment 50% of the shift on day one, 60% on day two, 80% on day three and 100% on day four. New CBP officers who will be similarly exposed should start with 20% on day one, with a 20% increase in exposure each additional day [NIOSH 1986]. The duration of exposure required for full acclimatization is highly variable between individuals, and some CBP officers may be able to work a full shift before this process is completed. The body's acclimatization will continue to improve each day in that hot environment for up to 3 weeks.

2. Develop inservice education programs to ensure that all CBP officers potentially exposed to hot environments stay current on heat stress and heat stress prevention information. CBP officers working in the outside inspection area should have inservice education at least yearly. An effective heat stress training program should include at least the following components:

   - knowledge of the hazards of heat stress

   - recognition of predisposing factors, danger signs, and symptoms

   - awareness of signs and symptoms of heat-related illness and first-aid procedures for treatment

   - CBP officer responsibilities in avoiding heat stress and informing their healthcare providers of their occupational exposures

- medical conditions that may increase the risk of heat-related illnesses

- information that certain prescription medications can interfere with the body's compensation mechanisms for heat stress and dehydration

- dangers in using drugs of any type (over-the-counter, prescription, or illicit) with stimulant properties, in hot and physically demanding work environments, as these substances increase the demand on the heart

- education of employees that alcoholic beverages will worsen dehydration in hot environments and should not be used for rehydration purposes

- preventive measures that can be taken to reduce heat stress

- encouraging CBP officers to take their breaks in a cool location such as the break room

3. Monitor environmental heat exposures during the hottest parts of the summer using a WBGT monitor at, or as close as possible to, the area where the CBP officers are exposed. CBP officers' break areas and other work areas may differ in temperature and should also be measured; results should be used to calculate hourly TWA WBGTs. Make at least hourly WBGT measurements during the hottest part of each shift, during the hottest parts of the year, and when heat waves occur or are predicted to occur. If two sequential measurements exceed the applicable recommendations (NIOSH RAL or REL, or ACGIH TLV), then work conditions should be modified until two more sequential WBGT measurements are within these exposure limits. On these days, administrative controls such as increasing the number of breaks and CBP officers in the inspection area, use of cooling methods, and additional awareness training can be implemented to help reduce the risk of heat-related illness.

4. Establish criteria for the declaration of a heat alert. For example, a heat alert may be declared if the area weather forecast for the next day predicts a maximum air temperature of 95°F or higher, or 90°F if this temperature is 9°F above the maximum reached in any of the preceding 3 days. Procedures to follow during the state of heat alert include:

- increasing the number of CBP officers in each team to reduce each employee's metabolic rate

- increasing rest allowances

- reminding CBP officers to drink small amounts of water frequently to prevent dehydration and maintain body weight, and to weigh themselves before and after the shift

- checking CBP officers' oral temperature and pulse during their most severe heat-exposure period

- exercising additional caution on the first day of a shift change to make sure CBP officers are not overexposed to heat, because they may have lost some of their acclimatization over the weekend and during days off

- restricting overtime work

5. Develop a heat-related illness surveillance program that includes establishing and maintaining accurate records of any heat-related disorder events and noting the environmental and work conditions at the time of disorder. Such events may include repeated accidents, episodes of heat-related disorders, or frequent health-related absences. Job-specific clustering of specific events or illnesses should be followed up by environmental and personal monitoring and medical evaluations.

6. Ensure that CBP officers stay hydrated and do not lose more than 1.5% body weight during their shift. Always provide cool (50°F–60°F) water or any cool liquid (except alcoholic beverages) and encourage CBP officers to drink small amounts frequently (e.g., one cup every 20 minutes). Drinking from individual containers improves water intake over the use of drinking fountains. Although some commercial drinks contain salt, this is not a necessary requirement because most people add enough salt to their diets to accommodate working in this environment.

7. Allow CBP officers to take unscheduled breaks if they report feeling weak, nauseated, excessively fatigued, confused, and/or irritable on days with high temperatures. Any individual experiencing loss of consciousness should be immediately transferred to the nearest emergency department for treatment of possible heat stroke, the most severe form of heat stress. These heat strain symptoms, and any other signs

RECOMMENDATIONS
(CONTINUED)

of heat overexposure, should be reported by CBP officers to their supervisor for investigation and follow-up.

The following recommendations can help reduce CO exposures and related illnesses in CBP officers.

1. Require all drivers entering the primary inspection area to turn off their vehicle when the CBP officer is inspecting the undercarriage. Turning off the vehicle will reduce peak exposures caused by the vehicle's exhaust. CBP officers indicated that vehicles are often left running because a large number fail to restart if they are shut off. If this remains a concern, CBP should evaluate having a tow truck on site to clear the stalled vehicle(s) from the inspection lane.

2. Develop a hazard communication program using the OSHA hazard communication standard as a program guideline. Sample programs can be found on the OSHA website at www.osha.gov/SLTC/hazardcommunications/index.html.

3. Continue CBP officer rotation even if it is not required for security reasons. The rotation acts as an administrative control by lowering the average CO exposure over a work shift.

4. Monitor CBP officers' CO exposure when changes in the workplace are made and compare these results with applicable OELs. Changes in ambient conditions, vehicle traffic, work practices, and a variety of other variables could greatly affect these results.

REFERENCES

NOAA [2000]. Climatography of the United States report No. 20: El Paso Intl AP, TX. Asheville, NC: U.S. Department of Commerce, National Oceanic and Atmospheric Administration, National Environmental Satellite, Data, and Information Service.

NIOSH [1986]. Criteria for a recommended standard: occupational exposure to hot environments, rev. Cincinnati, OH: U.S. Department of Health and Human Services, Centers for Disease Control, National Institute for Occupational Safety and Health, DHHS (NIOSH) Publication No. 86-113.

Heat Stress

We evaluated the heat stress conditions in the outside vehicle inspection areas by collecting WBGT measurements using four QUESTemp°36 instruments (Quest Technologies, Inc., Oconomowoc, Wisconsin). These monitors measure temperatures of 23°F–212°F and are accurate to within ± 0.9°F. In addition to temperature, the monitors measure relative humidity of 0%–100% and are accurate to within ± 5%. The WBGT index accounts for air velocity, temperature, humidity, and radiant heat and is a useful index of the environmental contribution to heat stress. WBGT is a function of dry bulb temperature (a standard measure of air temperature taken with a thermometer), natural wet bulb temperature (simulates the effects of evaporative cooling), and black globe temperature (estimates radiant [infrared] heat load). The WBGT monitors were placed throughout the primary and secondary vehicle inspection areas and in the head house. The monitors were set up to data log continuously. WBGT measurements were collected to document the heat stress conditions during the time that heat strain monitoring was conducted. Appendix B contains a discussion of occupational exposure limits and the health effects of working in hot environments.

Heat Strain

We assessed CBP officers' heat strain by collecting CBT measurements using the CorTemp™ Wireless Core Body Temperature Monitoring System (HQ, Inc., Palmetto, Florida). The CorTemp Temperature Sensor is swallowed and provides continuous monitoring of CBT to within ± 0.2°F. The sensor, intended for one-time use only, is passed through the gastrointestinal tract and exits the body in an average time of 72 hours. The sensor transmits the temperature to the CT2000 data logger. The participants' CBTs were recorded at 1-minute intervals.

We also assessed heat strain by collecting heart rate measurements using the Mini-Mitter Mini-Logger® Series 2000 (Mini-Mitter Company, Inc., Bend, Oregon) with a Polar® chest band heart rate monitor. The Polar chest band heart rate monitor counts up to 250 bpm and is accurate to within ± 1 bpm. Heart rate was monitored at 1-minute intervals.

We measured participants' preshift and postshift body weights to determine their degree of dehydration. Participants were weighed in uniform clothing near the beginning and end of the work shift using a self-calibrating electronic digital scale Model 812 (Measurement Specialties, Inc., Fairfield, New Jersey).

Following informed consent, preshift and postshift blood chemistry levels and hematology quantities were measured using the i-STAT® handheld analyzer, with i-STAT 8+ cartridges. Blood chemistries included serum sodium, potassium, chloride, BUN, and glucose. Hemoglobin and hematocrit (number of red blood cells per volume of blood) were also measured. Dehydration results in an increase in serum sodium, BUN, and hematocrit, whereas hyperhydration results in their decrease. Whole blood (65–95 microliters) was placed in the well of the cartridge prior to inserting the cartridge into the analyzer. Serum osmolality, dissolved particle concentration in the blood, is measured in mosm/L and was calculated from the blood chemistries using the following formula [Wallach 2000].

$$\text{osmolality} = (1.86 \times \text{serum sodium}) + \left(\frac{\text{serum glucose}}{18} \right) + \left(\frac{\text{BUN}}{2.8} \right)$$

A corrected serum sodium must be calculated for persons with elevated glucose levels because high serum glucose (> 100 mg/dL) can cause measurements of serum sodium to be falsely low. The formula for the corrected serum sodium is:

$$\text{corrected serum sodium} = \text{measured serum sodium} + \left(\frac{1.6 \times (\text{glucose} - 100)}{100} \right)$$

All participants completed a short heat stress questionnaire at the postshift assessment. This questionnaire included questions on medical history, possible heat stress symptoms, and factors that would affect acclimatization.

Carbon Monoxide

We assessed participants' CO exposure by collecting PBZ air measurements using Toxi Ultra single gas detectors (Biosystems, Middletown, Connecticut). These detectors data log the CO levels in real time at 1-minute intervals. The full shift TWA exposure and peak exposures were calculated. The detectors use an electrochemical cell to detect CO levels and were calibrated daily on site prior to use. The detectors are capable of measuring CO levels of 0–1,000 ppm; the generally accepted accuracy of electrochemical sensors is ± 5% or ± 2 ppm, whichever is greater. Potential interfering compounds found in vehicular exhaust include sulfur dioxide, nitrogen dioxide, nitric oxide, and hydrogen.

We also conducted biological monitoring to assess employees' CO exposure over the course of their shift. We used the MicroCO Meter (Micro Medical Limited, Rochester, Kent, United Kingdom) to measure CO in exhaled breath. The MicroCO Meter then calculates a corresponding %COHb that can be compared with the ACGIH BEI for COHb. The %COHb is used as a biological indicator of CO exposure. Before and after the shift we asked employees to inhale, then exhale completely, and then inhale deeply and hold their breath for 20 seconds. At the end of 20 seconds the employee exhaled through a one-way valve on the MicroCO Meter over an electrochemical sensor. By looking at the difference between preshift and postshift %COHb levels, we were able to determine the change over the shift, irrespective of employee smoking status.

Reference

Wallach J [2000]. Core blood analytes: alterations by diseases. In: Wallach J, ed. Interpretation of diagnostic tests, 7th ed. Philadelphia, PA: Lippincott, Williams and Wilkins, pp. 68-69.

In evaluating the hazards posed by workplace exposures, NIOSH investigators use both mandatory (legally enforceable) and recommended OELs for chemical, physical, and biological agents as a guide for making recommendations. OELs have been developed by Federal agencies and safety and health organizations to prevent the occurrence of adverse health effects from workplace exposures. Generally, OELs suggest levels of exposure to which most employees may be exposed up to 10 hours per day, 40 hours per week for a working lifetime without experiencing adverse health effects. However, not all employees will be protected from adverse health effects even if their exposures are maintained below these levels. A small percentage may experience adverse health effects because of individual susceptibility, a preexisting medical condition, and/or a hypersensitivity (allergy). In addition, some hazardous substances may act in combination with other workplace exposures, the general environment, or with medications or personal habits of the employee to produce health effects even if the occupational exposures are controlled at the level set by the exposure limit. Also, some substances can be absorbed by direct contact with the skin and mucous membranes in addition to being inhaled, which contributes to the individual's overall exposure.

Most OELs are expressed as a TWA exposure. A TWA refers to the average exposure during a normal 8- to 10-hour workday. Some chemical substances and physical agents have recommended STEL or ceiling values where health effects are caused by exposures over a short period. Unless otherwise noted, the STEL is a 15-minute TWA exposure that should not be exceeded at any time during a workday, and the ceiling limit is an exposure that should not be exceeded at any time.

In the United States, OELs have been established by Federal agencies, professional organizations, state and local governments, and other entities. Some OELs are legally enforceable limits, while others are recommendations. The U.S. Department of Labor OSHA PELs (29 CFR 1910 [general industry]; 29 CFR 1926 [construction industry]; and 29 CFR 1917 [maritime industry]) are legal limits enforceable in workplaces covered under the Occupational Safety and Health Act. NIOSH RELs are recommendations based on a critical review of the scientific and technical information available on a given hazard and the adequacy of methods to identify and control the hazard. NIOSH RELs can be found in the *NIOSH Pocket Guide to Chemical Hazards* [NIOSH 2005]. NIOSH also recommends different types of risk management practices (e.g., engineering controls, safe work practices, employee education/training, personal protective equipment, and exposure and medical monitoring) to minimize the risk of exposure and adverse health effects from these hazards. Other OELs that are commonly used and cited in the United States include the TLVs recommended by ACGIH, a professional organization, and the WEELs recommended by the American Industrial Hygiene Association, another professional organization. The TLVs and WEELs are developed by committee members of these associations from a review of the published, peer-reviewed literature. They are not consensus standards. ACGIH TLVs are considered voluntary exposure guidelines for use by industrial hygienists and others trained in this discipline "to assist in the control of health hazards" [ACGIH 2008a]. WEELs have been established for some chemicals "when no other legal or authoritative limits exist" [AIHA 2008].

Outside the United States, OELs have been established by various agencies and organizations and include both legal and recommended limits. Since 2006, the Berufsgenossenschaftliches Institut für Arbeitsschutz (German Institute for Occupational Safety and Health) has maintained a database of international OELs from European Union member states, Canada (Québec), Japan, Switzerland, and the United States at www.dguv.de/bgia/en/gestis/limit_values/index.jsp. The database contains international limits for over 1250 hazardous substances and is updated annually.

Employers should understand that not all hazardous chemicals have specific OSHA PELs, and for some agents the legally enforceable and recommended limits may not reflect current health-based information. However, an employer is still required by OSHA to protect its employees from hazards even in the absence of a specific OSHA PEL. OSHA requires an employer to furnish employees a place of employment free from recognized hazards that cause or are likely to cause death or serious physical harm [Occupational Safety and Health Act of 1970 (Public Law 91–596, sec. 5(a)(1))]. Thus, NIOSH investigators encourage employers to make use of other OELs when making risk assessment and risk management decisions to best protect the health of their employees. NIOSH investigators also encourage the use of the traditional hierarchy of controls approach to eliminate or minimize identified workplace hazards. This includes, in order of preference, the use of: (1) substitution or elimination of the hazardous agent, (2) engineering controls (e.g., local exhaust ventilation, process enclosure, dilution ventilation), (3) administrative controls (e.g , limiting time of exposure, employee training, work practice changes, medical surveillance), and (4) personal protective equipment (e.g., respiratory protection, gloves, eye protection, hearing protection). Control banding, a qualitative risk assessment and risk management tool, is a complementary approach to protecting employee health that focuses resources on exposure controls by describing how a risk needs to be managed. Additional information on control banding is available at www.cdc.gov/niosh/topics/ctrlbanding/. This approach can be applied in situations where OELs have not been established or can be used to supplement the OELs, when available.

Heat Stress

NIOSH defines heat stress exposure as the sum of the heat generated in the body (metabolic heat) plus the heat gained from the environment (environmental heat) minus the heat lost from the body to the environment, primarily through evaporation. Many bodily responses to heat stress are desirable and beneficial because they help regulate internal temperature and, in situations of appropriate repeated exposure, help the body adapt (acclimatize) to the work environment. However, at some stage of heat stress, the body's compensatory measures cannot maintain internal body temperature at the level required for normal functioning. As a result, the risk of heat-induced illnesses, disorders, and accidents substantially increases. Increases in unsafe behavior, behavior that may lead to accidents, are also seen as the level of physical work of the job increases [NIOSH 1986].

Many heat stress guidelines have been developed to protect people against heat-related illnesses. The objective of any heat stress index is to prevent a person's CBT from rising excessively. The World Health Organization concluded that, "it is inadvisable for CBT to exceed 100.4°F or for oral temperature to exceed 99.5°F in prolonged daily exposure to heavy work and/or heat" [WHO 1969]. According to NIOSH, a CBT of 102.2°F should be considered reason to terminate exposure even when CBT is being monitored. This does not mean that an employee with a CBT exceeding those levels will necessarily experience adverse health effects; however, the number of unsafe acts increases as does the risk of developing heat stress illnesses [NIOSH 1986]. A CBT increase of only 1.8°F above normal encroaches on the brain's ability to function [ACGIH 2008a].

NIOSH recommends controlling total heat exposure so that unprotected healthy employees who are medically and physically fit for their required level of activity are wearing, at most, long-sleeved work shirts and trousers or equivalent, and are not exposed to metabolic and environmental heat combinations exceeding the applicable NIOSH recommendations. Most healthy employees who work in hot environments and are exposed to combinations of environmental and metabolic heat less than the NIOSH RALs for nonacclimatized employees, or the NIOSH RELs for acclimatized employees, should be able to tolerate total heat stress without substantially increasing their risk of incurring acute adverse health effects. Also, no employee should be exposed to combinations of metabolic and environmental heat exceeding the applicable ceiling limits shown in Figures 1 or 2 without being provided with and properly using appropriate and adequate heat-protective clothing and equipment [NIOSH 1986].

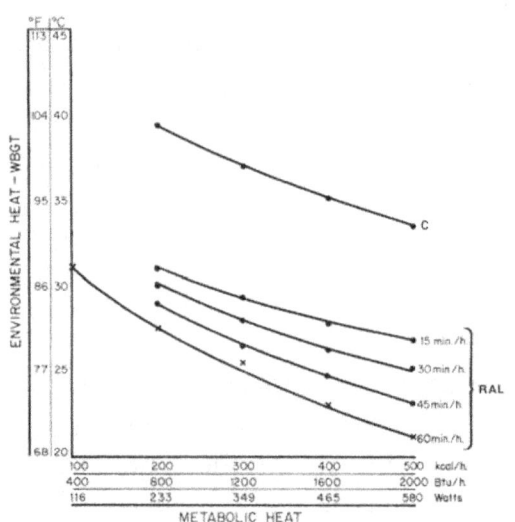

Figure 1. Recommended heat-stress alert limits (unacclimatized employees).

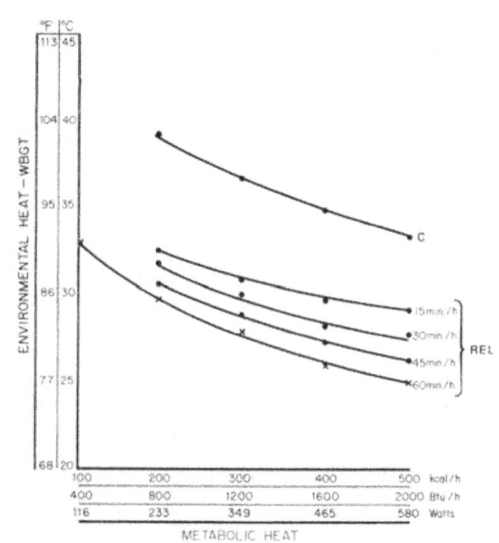

Figure 2. Recommended heat-stress limits (acclimatized employees).

ACGIH guidelines require the use of a decision-making process that provides step-by-step situation-dependent instructions that factor in clothing insulation values and physiological evaluation of heat strain [ACGIH 2008b]. ACGIH WBGT screening recommendations factor in the ability of the body to cool itself (clothing insulation value, humidity, and wind) and, like the NIOSH recommendations, can be used to develop work/rest regimens for employees. The ACGIH WBGT-based heat exposure assessment was developed for a traditional work uniform of long-sleeved shirt and pants, and represents conditions under which it is believed that nearly all adequately hydrated, unmedicated, healthy employees may be repeatedly exposed without adverse health effects. Clothing insulation values and the appropriate WBGT adjustments, as well as descriptors of the other decision-making process components can be found in ACGIH's *Documentation of the Threshold Limit Values for Chemical Substances and Physical Agents and Biological Exposure Indices* [ACGIH 2008b]. The ACGIH TLV for heat stress provides a framework for the control of heat-related illnesses only. Although accidents and injuries can increase with increasing levels of heat stress, the TLVs are not directed toward controlling these [ACGIH 2008a].

NIOSH and ACGIH recommendations can only be used when WBGT data for the immediate work area are available and must not be used when employees wear encapsulating suits or garments that are impermeable or highly resistant to water vapor or air movement. Further assumptions regarding work demands include an 8-hour work day, 5-day work week, two 15-minute breaks, and a 30-minute lunch break, with rest area temperatures the same as, or less than, those in work areas, and at least some air movement. It must be stressed that because NIOSH and ACGIH guidelines do not establish a fine line between safe and dangerous levels, professional judgment must be used in administering a heat stress management program to ensure adequate protection. The OSHA technical manual's section on heat stress refers back to the ACGIH document for guidelines to evaluate employee heat stress and how to investigate the workplace [OSHA 1999].

Heat Strain

The body's response to heat stress is called heat strain [NIOSH 1986; ACGIH 2008b]. Operations involving high air temperatures, radiant heat sources, high humidity, direct physical contact with hot objects, and strenuous physical activities have a high potential for inducing heat strain in employees. Heat strain is highly individual and cannot be predicted based upon environmental heat stress measurements. Physiological monitoring for heat strain becomes necessary when impermeable clothing is worn, when heat stress recommendations are exceeded, or when data from a detailed analysis (such as the International Standards Organization required sweat rate) shows excess heat stress [ACGIH 2008b].

One indicator of physiological strain, sustained peak heart rate, is considered by ACGIH to be the best sign of acute, high-level exposure to heat stress. Sustained peak heart rate, defined by ACGIH as 180 bpm minus an individual's age, is a leading indicator that thermal regulatory control may not be adequate and that increases in CBTs have, or will soon, occur. Sustained peak heart rate represents an equivalent cardiovascular demand of about 75% of maximum aerobic capacity. During an 8-hour workshift, although sustained peak demands may not occur, excessive demand may still be placed on the cardiovascular system. These 'chronic' demands can be measured by calculating the average heart rate over the shift [ACGIH 2008b]. A study of Marine Corps recruits revealed that decreases in physical job performance were observed when the average heart rate exceeded 115 bpm over the entire shift. This level is equivalent to working at roughly 35% of maximum aerobic capacity, a level sustainable for 8 hours [Minard 1961].

According to ACGIH, an individual's heat stress exposure should be discontinued when *any* of the following excessive heat strain indicators occur:

- Sustained (over several minutes) heart rate is in excess of 180 bpm minus the individual's age in years, (180 bpm – age) for those with normal cardiac performance

- CBT is greater than 100.4°F for unselected, unacclimatized personnel and greater than 101.3°F for medically fit, heat-acclimatized personnel

- Recovery heart rate at 1 minute after a peak work effort exceeds 110 bpm

- Symptoms of sudden and severe fatigue, nausea, dizziness, or lightheadedness

An individual may be at greater risk of heat strain if:

- Profuse sweating is sustained over several hours

- Weight loss over a shift is greater than 1 5% of body weight

- 24-hour urinary sodium excretion is less than 55 millimoles

Health Effects of Exposure to Hot Environments

Heat disorders and health effects of individuals exposed to hot working environments include (in increasing order of severity) skin disorders (heat rash, hives, etc.), heat syncope (fainting), heat cramps, heat exhaustion, and heat stroke. Heat syncope results from blood flow being directed to the skin for cooling, resulting in decreased supply to the brain, and most often strikes employees who stand in place for extended periods in hot environments. Heat cramps, caused by sodium depletion due to sweating, typically occur in the muscles employed in strenuous work. Heat cramps and syncope often accompany heat exhaustion, or weakness, fatigue, confusion, nausea, and other symptoms. The dehydration, sodium loss, and elevated CBT (above 100.4°F) are usually due to performing strenuous work in hot conditions with inadequate water and electrolyte intake. Heat exhaustion may lead to heat stroke if the patient is not quickly cooled and rehydrated.

While heat exhaustion victims continue to sweat as their bodies struggle to stay cool, heat stroke victims cease to sweat as their bodies fail to maintain an appropriate core temperature. Heat stroke occurs when hard work, hot environment, and dehydration overload the body's cooling capacity. Heat stroke is a life-threatening emergency requiring immediate medical attention. Signs and symptoms include irritability, confusion, nausea, convulsions or unconsciousness, hot dry skin, and a CBT above 106°F. Death can result from damage to the brain, heart, liver, or kidneys [Cohen 1990].

Prolonged increases in CBT and chronic exposures to high levels of heat stress are associated with disorders such as temporary infertility (male and female), elevated heart rate, sleep disturbance, fatigue, and irritability. During the first trimester of pregnancy, a sustained CBT greater than 102.2°F may endanger the fetus [ACGIH 2008a]. In addition, one or more occurrences of heat-induced illness in a person predisposes him/her to subsequent injuries and can result in temporary or permanent loss of that person's ability to tolerate heat stress [NIOSH 1986; OSHA 1999].

The level of heat stress at which health effects occur is highly individual and depends upon the heat tolerance capabilities of each individual. Age, weight, degree of physical fitness, degree of acclimatization, metabolism, alcohol or illicit drugs, over-the-counter and prescribed medications, and a variety of medical conditions, such as hypertension and diabetes, all affect a person's sensitivity to heat. At greatest risk are unacclimatized employees, people performing physically strenuous work, those with previous heat illnesses, the elderly, people with cardiovascular or circulatory disorders (diabetes, atherosclerotic vascular disease), those taking medications that impair the body's cooling mechanisms, people who use alcohol or who used it recently, people in poor physical condition, and those recovering from illness. Prescribed medications such as beta blockers and calcium-channel blockers, which are used to treat hypertension, limit maximal cardiac output and alter normal vascular distribution of blood flow in response to heat exposure. Diuretics, such as alcohol, can limit cardiac output and affect heat tolerance and sweating; antihistamines, phenothiazines, and cyclic antidepressants can impair sweating.

Acclimatization

When employees are first exposed to a hot environment, they show signs of distress and discomfort, experience increased CBTs and heart rates, and may have headaches and/or nausea. Repeated exposure results in marked adaptation to the hot environment known as acclimatization. Acclimatization is the process that allows the body to begin sweating sooner and more efficiently, reduces electrolyte concentrations in the sweat, and allows the circulation to stabilize so that the employee can withstand greater amounts of heat stress while experiencing reduced heat strain signs and symptoms.

Acclimatization begins with consecutive exposures to working conditions for 2 hours at a time, with a requisite rise in metabolic rate. This will cause the body to reach 33% of optimum acclimatization by the fourth day of exposure. Cardiovascular function will stabilize, and surface and internal body temperatures will be lower by day 8 when the body has reached 44% of optimum acclimatization. A decrease in sweat and urine electrolyte concentrations is seen at 65% of optimum (day 10); 93% of optimum is reached by day 18, and 99% by day 21 [ACGIH 2008b].

The loss of acclimatization begins when the activity under those heat stress conditions is discontinued, and a noticeable loss occurs after 4 days. This loss is usually rapidly made up so that by Tuesday, employees who were off on the weekend are as well acclimatized as they were on the preceding Friday. Chronic illness, an acute episode of mild illness (e.g., gastroenteritis), the use or misuse of pharmacologic agents, a sleep deficit, a suboptimal nutritional state, or a disturbed water and electrolyte balance may reduce the employee's capacity to acclimatize [ACGIH 2008b].

Dehydration and Hyponatremia

When working in hot environments it is often difficult to completely replace lost fluids as the day's work proceeds. High sweat rates with excessive loss of body fluids may result in dehydration and electrolyte imbalances [Bates et al. 1996]. Some studies have shown that even small deficits adversely affect performance [Sawka et al. 1993]. Dehydration also negates the advantage granted by high levels of aerobic fitness and heat acclimatization [Ekblom et al. 1970].

Several studies have shown that dehydration increases CBT during exercise in temperate and hot environments; a deficit of only 1% of body weight increases CBT during exercise. As the magnitude of the water deficit increases, an accompanying elevation in CBT occurs when exercising in the heat. The magnitude of this elevation ranges from 0.2°F–0.4°F for every 1% body weight loss [Sawka et al. 1979]. A 2% loss of body weight is generally accepted as the threshold for thirst stimulation [Szlyk et al. 1989]. A 3% decrease in body weight causes an increase in heart rate, depressed sweating sensitivity, and a substantial decrease in physical work capacity [Candas et al. 1986]. Some investigators have reported that a 4%–6% water deficit has been associated with anorexia, impatience, and headache, while a 6%–10% deficit is associated with vertigo, shortness of breath, cyanosis, and spasticity. With a 12% water deficit, an individual will be unable to swallow and will need assistance with rehydration. Body weight loss of 1 5% or less indicates mild dehydration, whereas a loss of greater than 1.5% indicates a greater risk of heat stress.

Because water is the most abundant constituent in the body, comprising approximately 60% of the body weight in men and 50% in women, maintaining enough water improves the body's overall function. Total body water is distributed in two major compartments: 55%–75% is intracellular fluid and 25%–45% is extracellular fluid [Singer and Brenner 1998]. The solute, or dissolved particle concentration of a fluid, is known as its osmolality, expressed as mosm/L. The major extracellular fluid component is sodium; therefore, extracellular fluid volume reflects total body sodium content.

Normal plasma osmolality ranges from 275–290 mosm/L and is kept within a narrow range by mechanisms capable of sensing a 1%–2% change in plasma concentration. Most people have an obligate water loss consisting of urine, stool, and evaporation from the skin and respiratory tract. In order to maintain a steady state, water intake must equal water excretion. Disorders of water regulation result in hyponatremia or hypernatremia. Changes in urine and plasma osmolality are better suited for diagnosing hydration status than changes in hematocrit, serum protein, and BUN, which are more dependent on factors other than hydration [Wallach 2000; ACGIH 2008a]. The primary stimulus for water ingestion is thirst, which can be triggered by the following physiological mechanisms: an increase in osmolality, a decrease in extracellular fluid volume, or a decrease in blood pressure. Osmoreceptors in the hypothalamus are stimulated by a rise in serum concentration. The average osmotic threshold for thirst is approximately 295 milliosmoles per kilogram and varies among individuals. Under normal circumstances, daily water intake exceeds physiological requirements [Rolls 1993].

In addition to dehydration, there is also the matter of electrolyte depletion as a factor in heat stress, Sodium, a vital electrolyte, is excreted as the body sweats in order to utilize evaporative cooling. Two of the many functions of sodium in the body are to conduct impulses along neurons and maintain concentration gradients in the kidney for proper urine production.

Most individuals with acute exercise-induced heat disorder are dehydrated with normal to mildly increased serum sodium and serum osmolality (hypernatremia). Hyponatremia develops when serum sodium levels drop below 135 mEq/L and is a life-threatening condition that has been recognized as a potential health consequence of endurance activities conducted in hot environments. Increased water intake prior to and during activities in hot environments is highly emphasized to prevent dehydration and heat illness. However, drinking too much water can lead to decreased serum sodium concentrations (water toxicity or hyponatremia) and has been recognized as an increasing problem among U.S. military recruits [Gardner 2002].

Hyponatremia may occur with hypo-, hyper-, or normal hydration status [Roetzheim 1991]. Symptomatic and potentially life-threating hyponatremia can occur when blood sodium concentrations decrease to less than 130 mEq/L and is generally caused by hypervolemia (water overload) secondary to extensive overdrinking. Many people with hyponatremia have increased their total body water by about 1 gallon to achieve such low serum sodium values [Montain et al. 1999].

Most cases of hyponatremia result from the inability of the kidneys to excrete appropriately diluted urine. The most significant clinical signs of hyponatremia involve the central nervous system, where symptoms vary from subtle changes in one's ability to think and decreases in energy levels to severe alterations, such as coma or seizure. Symptoms generally parallel the rate of development and degree of hyponatremia [Devita 1993].

Fluid Replacement

Palatability of any fluid replacement solution is important to ensure adequate rehydration. Evidence shows that adding sweeteners to drinks leads to increased consumption. Glucose-electrolyte solutions have been shown to facilitate sodium and water absorption. Also, the glucose in these solutions provides energy for muscular activity in endurance events that require vigorous exercise [Rolls 1990]. However, employees should be cautioned to avoid drinking large amounts of sugar-laden beverages in hot climates as this causes an osmotic diuresis that increases fluid loss through urination. Alcohol intake also increase urinary fluid loss and should be avoided. The temperature of the drink also influences consumption of fluids. Ideally, fluids should be ingested at temperatures of 50°F–60°F, in small quantities (5–7 ounces), and at frequent intervals (every 15–20 minutes).

Average Americans consume adequate, if not excessive, amounts of sodium in their usual diet such that for mild dehydration, only water replacement is needed. However, in moderate dehydration or when involved in events resulting in prolonged sweating, electrolyte (i.e., sodium) replacement is indicated. Many oral electrolyte replacement formulas such as Gatorade® are available. Salt tablets are not recommended as they can irritate the stomach, leading to vomiting, which can exacerbate fluid losses and do not address water replacement needs. Those with nausea and vomiting from heat stress may require intravenous saline administration to replace their water and sodium.

Carbon Monoxide

CO is a colorless, odorless, tasteless gas produced by incomplete burning of carbon-containing materials such as gasoline or propane fuel. The initial symptoms of CO poisoning may include headache, dizziness, drowsiness, or nausea. Symptoms may advance to vomiting, loss of consciousness, and collapse if prolonged or high exposures are encountered. If the exposure level is high, loss of consciousness may occur without any other symptoms. Coma or death may occur if high exposures continue. The display of symptoms varies widely from individual to individual and may occur sooner in susceptible individuals such as young or aged people, people with pre-existing lung or heart disease, or those living at high altitudes.

Exposure to CO limits the ability of the blood to carry oxygen to the tissues by occupying the oxygen binding sites on hemoglobin to form COHb. Once absorbed in the bloodstream, the half life (time it takes for half of the substance to be removed) of CO disappearance from the blood varies widely by individual and circumstance (e.g., removal from exposure, initial COHb concentration, partial pressure of oxygen after exposure, etc.). Under normal recovery conditions breathing ambient air, the expected half life is approximately 5 hours [Tomaszewski 2002].

The OSHA PEL for CO is 50 ppm for an 8-hour TWA exposure. The NIOSH REL for CO is 35 ppm for a 10-hour TWA exposure, with a ceiling of 200 ppm that should not be exceeded [NIOSH 1992]. The NIOSH REL is designed to protect employees from health effects associated with COHb levels that exceed 5% [NIOSH 1972]. NIOSH has established the IDLH for CO as 1,200 ppm. The IDLH exposure conditions pose "a threat of exposure to airborne contaminants when that exposure is likely to cause death or immediate or delayed permanent adverse health effects or prevent escape from such an environment" [NIOSH 2004].

ACGIH recommends an 8-hour TWA TLV of 25 ppm based upon limiting shifts in COHb levels to less than 3.5%, thus minimizing adverse neurobehavioral changes such as headache, dizziness, etc., and to maintain cardiovascular exercise capacity [ACGIH 2008a]. ACGIH also recommends that exposures never exceed five times the TLV (thus, never to exceed 125 ppm) [ACGIH 2008b]. ACGIH recommends a BEI for end of shift COHb in blood of 3 5% [ACGIH 2008a]. The BEI indicates a concentration below which nearly all employees should not experience adverse health effects. The BEI cannot be applied to current smokers because they have been shown to have COHb levels between 4% and 10%, and can exceed 15% in heavy smokers [ACGIH 2008a; Tomaszewski 2002]. The World Health Organization established the reference ranges for COHb between 1%–2% for nonsmokers and 3%–8% for smokers [WHO 1999].

References

ACGIH [2008a]. 2008 TLVs® and BEIs®: threshold limit values for chemical substances and physical agents and biological exposure indices. Cincinnati, OH: American Conference of Governmental Industrial Hygienists.

ACGIH [2008b]. Documentation of the threshold limit values and biological exposure indices. 7th ed. Cincinnati, OH: American Conference of Governmental Industrial Hygienists; 2002–2008 Suppl.

AIHA [2008]. AIHA 2008 Emergency response planning guidelines (ERPG) & workplace environmental exposure levels (WEEL) handbook. Fairfax, VA: American Industrial Hygiene Association.

Bates G, Gazey C, Cena K [1996]. Factors affecting heat illness when working in conditions of thermal stress. J Hum Ergon 25(1):13–20.

Candas V, Libert JP, Brandenberger G, Sagot JC, Amoros C, Kahn JM [1986]. Hydration during exercise: effects on thermal and cardiovascular adjustments. Eur J Appl Physiol 55(2):113–122.

CFR. Code of Federal Regulations. Washington, DC: U.S. Government Printing Office, Office of the Federal Register.

Cohen R [1990]. Injuries due to physical hazards. In: LaDou J, ed. Occupational medicine. East Norwalk, CT: Appleton & Lange.

DeVita MV, Michelis MF [1993]. Perturbations in sodium balance, hyponatremia and hypernatremia. Clin Lab Med 13(1):135–148.

Ekblom B, Greenleaf CJ, Greenleaf JE, Hermansen L [1970]. Temperature regulation during exercise dehydration in man. Acta Physiol Scand 79(4):475–483.

Gardner JW [2002]. Death by water intoxication. Mil Med 167:502–508.

Minard D [1961]. Prevention of heat casualties in Marine Corps recruits. Period of 1955-60, with comparative incidence rates and climatic heat stresses in other training categories. Mil Med 126:261–272.

Montain SJ, Latzka WA, Sawka MN [1999]. Fluid replacement recommendations for training in hot weather. Mil Med 164(7):502–508.

NIOSH [1972]. Criteria for a recommended standard: occupational exposure to carbon monoxide. Cincinnati, OH: U.S. Department of Health, Education, and Welfare, Health Services and Mental Health Administration, National Institute for Occupational Safety and Health, DHEW (NIIOSH) Publication No. HSM 73-11000.

NIOSH [1986]. Criteria for a recommended standard: occupational exposure to hot environments, rev. Cincinnati, OH: U.S. Department of Health and Human Services, Centers for Disease Control, National Institute for Occupational Safety and Health, DHHS (NIOSH) Publication No. 86-113.

NIOSH [1992]. Recommendations for occupational safety and health: compendium of policy documents and statements. Cincinnati, OH: U.S. Department of Health and Human Services, Centers for Disease Control and Prevention, National Institute for Occupational Safety and Health, DHHS (NIOSH) Publication No. 92-100.

NIOSH [2004]. NIOSH Respirator Decision Logic. Cincinnati, OH: U.S. Department of Health and Human Services, Public Health Service, Centers for Disease Control and Prevention, National Institute for Occupational Safety and Health, DHHS (NIOSH) Publication No. 87-108.

NIOSH [2005]. NIOSH pocket guide to chemical hazards. Cincinnati, OH: U.S. Department of Health and Human Services, Centers for Disease Control and Prevention, National Institute for Occupational Safety and Health, DHHS (NIOSH) Publication No. 2005-149.

OSHA [1999]. Heat stress. In: OSHA technical manual. Sec 3 Chap 4. Washington, DC, U.S. Department of Labor, Occupational Safety and Health Administration, TED 1-0.15A.

Roetzheim R [1991]. Overhydration. Physician Sports Med 19(2):32.

Rolls BJ, Kim S, Federoff IC [1990]. Effects of drinks sweetened with sucrose or aspartame on hunger, thirst and food intake in men. Physiol Behav 48(1):19–26.

Rolls BJ [1993]. Palatability and fluid intake. In: Mariott BM, ed. Fluid replacement and heat stress. Washington DC: National Academy Press, pp. 161–167.

Sawka MN, Knowlton RG, Critz JB [1979]. The thermal and circulatory responses to repeated bouts of prolonged running. Med Sci Sports 11(2):177–180.

Sawka MN, Neufer PD [1993]. Interaction of water bioavailability, thermoregulation, and exercise performance. In: Marriott BM, ed. Fluid replacement and heat stress. Washington DC: National Academy Press, pp. 85–95.

Singer GG, Brenner BM [1998]. Fluid and electrolyte disturbances. In: Fauci AS, Brunwald E, Isselbacher KJ, Wilson JD, Martin JB, Kasper DL, Hauser SL, Longo DL, eds. Harrison's principles of internal medicine, 14th ed. New York: Mc-Graw Hill.

Szlyk PC, Sils IV, Francesconi RP, Hubbard RW, Mattew WT [1989]. Variability in intake and dehydration in young men during a simulated desert walk. Aviat Space Environ Med 60(5):422–427.

Tomaszewski C [2002]. Carbon monoxide. In: Goldfrank LR. Goldfrank's toxicologic emergencies 7th Edition, New York: McGraw Hill, pp. 1478–1497.

Wallach J [2000]. Core blood analytes: alterations by diseases. In: Wallach J, ed. Interpretation of diagnostic tests, 7th ed. Philadelphia, PA: Lippincott Williams and Wilkins, pp. 68–69.

WHO [1969]. Health factors involved in working under conditions of heat stress. Geneva, Switzerland: World Health Organization. Technical Report Series No. 412.

WHO [1999]. Environmental Health Criteria 213–carbon monoxide (Second Edition). World Health Organization, Geneva. ISBN 92 4 157213 2 (NLM Classification: QV 662) ISSN 0250-863X.

ACKNOWLEDGMENTS AND AVAILABILITY OF REPORT

The Hazard Evaluations and Technical Assistance Branch (HETAB) of the National Institute for Occupational Safety and Health (NIOSH) conducts field investigations of possible health hazards in the workplace. These investigations are conducted under the authority of Section 20(a)(6) of the Occupational Safety and Health Administration (OSHA) Act of 1970, 29 U.S.C. 669(a)(6) which authorizes the Secretary of Health and Human Services, following a written request from any employer or authorized representative of employees, to determine whether any substance normally found in the place of employment has potentially toxic effects in such concentrations as used or found. HETAB also provides, upon request, technical and consultative assistance to federal, state, and local agencies; labor; industry; and other groups or individuals to control occupational health hazards and to prevent related trauma and disease.

The findings and conclusions in this report are those of the authors and do not necessarily represent the views of NIOSH. Mention of any company or product does not constitute endorsement by NIOSH. In addition, citations to websites external to NIOSH do not constitute NIOSH endorsement of the sponsoring organization or their programs or products. Furthermore, NIOSH is not responsible for the content of these websites. All Web addresses referenced in this document were accessible as of the publication date.

This report was prepared by Chad H. Dowell and Judith Eisenberg of HETAB, Division of Surveillance, Hazard Evaluations and Field Studies (DSHEFS). Industrial hygiene field assistance was provided by Brad King. Medical field assistance was provided by Sang Woo Tak. Health communication assistance was provided by Stefanie Evans. Editorial assistance was provided by Ellen Galloway. Desktop publishing was performed by Robin Smith.

Copies of this report have been sent to employee and management representatives at the U.S. Customs and Border Protection, the state health department, and the OSHA Regional Office. This report is not copyrighted and may be freely reproduced. The report may be viewed and printed from www.cdc.gov/niosh/hhe. Copies may be purchased from the National Technical Information Service (NTIS) at 5825 Port Royal Road, Springfield, Virginia 22161.